A Journey to Healing

5 Stages to Achieving More Freedom in Your Health and Your Life

LEONA ALLEN, D.C., PSc.D

BALBOA. PRESS
A DIVISION OF HAY HOUSE

Balboa Press books may be ordered through booksellers or by contacting:

Balboa Press
A Division of Hay House
1663 Liberty Drive
Bloomington, IN 47403
www.balboapress.com
1 (877) 407-4847

Print information available on the last page.

ISBN: 978-1-5043-2599-8 (sc)
ISBN: 978-1-5043-2601-8 (hc)
ISBN: 978-1-5043-2600-1 (e)

Library of Congress Control Number: 2014922997

Balboa Press rev. date: 3/2/2015

To my mother, my greatest inspiration and biggest fan. She is on a new journey now, and her spirit lives on in me and those she loved. I love you, Mom, and thank you for being a part of my journey.

Contents

Preface

This book illustrates the stages we must all go through in order to achieve more freedom in our health and in our lives. I am forever grateful for my journey, which has allowed me to be a better doctor, wife, friend, and mother. It is also a journey that has inspired me to write this book.

If you are struggling with any aspect of your health or if you are thinking that you are prone to some awful disease because it runs in the family, let that belief system go. You are not doomed for cancer or heart disease because your mother or father had it. If you start to disown your illness now, you are already on your way to healing.

I would love to hear about your journey. Please share your stories at www.DrLeona.com. Also, visit the website for more resources and tools that will help you along your journey.

Here's to your journey, and I am honored to be a part of it.

In health and in freedom,
Dr. Leona

Foreword

This book is a unique answer to the greatest problem faced by those looking to stick to a diet or lifestyle change. It is not just the answer to why you may have failed in the past with a diet or weight loss plan, but it also gives you strategies that you need to finally achieve success.

Most fail not because of the lack of desire to change but because of the lack of an understanding of how the human brain resists change, even change that can potentially save lives.

What if you knew in advance of a predictable but irrational process your brain will go through that has led to past failures in your journey to health and healing? If you knew ahead of time, you would not be surprised at your brain's seemingly irrational thoughts of sabotage and instead respond not out of guilt or defeat but from an offensive stance that causes a different outcome.

I believe *A Journey to Healing* is an answer to the prayers of so many who have failed in the past. *A Journey to Healing* walks you through the five phases every human brain goes through in the battle to change your lifestyle as well as gives you the answers to overcome and not repeat past processes.

As a practitioner, I have walked hundreds, if not thousands, of people through this battle, and when I read this book, I was captivated by how Dr. Leona, in a simple story format, put into words what I have seen over and over again. I was amazed at how she not only walked us through the struggle but also gave the reader clever answers for success.

As I read the book, my mind kept thinking of people who needed or need to read this. It is no doubt a game changer in the area of breakthrough that so many desire and need yet have fallen short of in the past.

A book is only as good or inspirational as the author who writes it, and I have found that it is only through the victories in the adversities and struggles in our own lives that give us the authority we need to make a difference in the lives of others. True to this fact, I believe it is Dr. Leona's own story and victories that make this book the real answer that it is. She is a doctor who understands what it is like to be sick, as well as battles the same temptations and setbacks that most of us face.

She has been and is an inspiration to so many suffering, and this book is a reflection of who she is and what God has called her to do.

Daniel Pompa, D.PSc.
Author of *The Cellular Healing Diet*

Introduction

Are you struggling with high blood pressure, diabetes, chronic fatigue, mood swings, muscle or joint pain, poor skin, digestive problems, or the inability to lose weight? Do you have trouble getting up in the morning and going to sleep at night and lack the energy and stamina that is required to function in between?

Are you taking medications? Are they helping you or hurting you? You may not even be on medications … you may be taking "natural" herbs and supplements from your local health food store and still lack the strength that you need to get through the day.

Are you searching for answers about what is really happening with your health and your body? Whatever the situation, the point is you are tired of feeling the way you are feeling and you want to know what you can do to fix it.

You may have already invested hundreds or even thousands of dollars on a healing program or protocol, whether it was from your own research or from the help of a specialist. As a result, did you feel better for a while and then your progress stopped? Did you end up feeling worse? Or did nothing appear to change at all?

Then what happened? Did you go on to the next program, supplement, medication, healer, product, or affirmation, and days to years later, are you still dealing with the same health challenges or maybe a few more? With this type of cycle, you become frustrated and end up losing hope. You begin to wonder if you have to live with it, but deep down inside, you don't want to give up. You still want to feel well, but you are tired of failing.

In our current information age, it is now more overwhelming than ever! With the internet and social media, when we have a problem, we use a search engine to research the topic and, voila, receive hundreds of different solutions mainly from complete strangers with questionable credentials. "Experts" are disagreeing with each other, and one fad replaces another. Wellness companies and products are everywhere, claiming to have the best product. Where do we go, and what do we do? Whom can we trust?

It becomes confusing and overwhelming. You've tried this thing and that thing. Some things seem to work, some don't. You hear this promise and that promise. One product works miraculously for your best friend but ends up making you completely sick. For example, say you and your friend shared a common long-term struggle with losing weight. She decided to try the latest weight-loss cleanse that involved meal-replacement shakes and nutritionals that help cleanse the liver and intestines. In fewer than thirty days, she lost twenty pounds and looked and felt amazing. So you quickly signed up, hoping to get similar results. Only days after starting the program, you experienced bloating, nausea, and diarrhea and immediately stopped the program, wondering what had happened. Was it your body or was the problem in the products? Frustrated, you concluded that cleanses don't work and decided to try something else or nothing at all.

Timing is another challenge. You wonder how long it will take you to get well. If your expectations aren't met and you don't see apparent results in seven to ten days, you quit and move on to the next thing or just give up altogether.

Other challenges involve believing that you are the only one with the problem and no one understands. Or intentionally or unintentionally believing that you don't deserve to be healthy and end up engaged in behavior that may sabotage your health.

Great health is our birthright. We all have the ability to heal.

But the reality is that healing, just like getting sick, is a process, and it takes time. And the timing it takes depends on you.

I've tried dozens of programs, and many of them did more harm than good. Since my early teens and into early adulthood, I have dealt with severe menstrual cramping, mood swings, skin breakouts, and frequent headaches. As I moved into my late thirties and early forties, I dealt with trouble losing weight and low energy. I would get rid of one symptom just to be welcomed by another. I have lost weight only to gain it back. I would give up and then start over again.

I've also discovered in my journey that being healthy is

beyond the right foods or supplements. It plays an important role, but we really have to incorporate the mind-set, the commitment, and the willingness to do whatever it takes in the right order and at the right time.

Despite the struggle and the frustration, I have overcome weight trouble, fatigue, depression, and hormonal issues and have helped others do the same. I've been through the ups and downs. I have turned my health and my life around, and you know what? You can too! I am at a healthy weight, and I feel stronger and more energetic than I ever did in my twenties. I enjoy running, dancing, and doing CrossFit.[1] My body is stronger, and I am stronger mentally as well. I have a more positive and proactive approach to life.

Achieving true health and wellness is similar to building a house, starting a business, or planning a trip. There are steps or stages involved. If you took a road trip from Georgia to California, you would prepare for the traffic jams, the hotel stays, and the pit stops and, with patience and perseverance, press on until you reach your destination. This is the most difficult part of making any real change; you *are* going to run into challenges and obstacles, and you *are* going to have successes as well as setbacks. Knowing what you are up against and having strategies to navigate challenges are what will ultimately lead you to reach your health goals.

Getting well is a process—a journey that involves the right mind-set, accurate information, and correct choices over time.

---

[1] "What is CrossFit?" CrossFit, accessed October 27, 2014, http://www.crossfit.com/cf-info/what-is-crossfit.html.

It involves experience, growth, and change. You are going to have good days and bad days, and there is *always* room for improvement.

It may be fair to say that you have this book in your hands right now because you are looking for a different approach. I am honored that you have chosen this book, and I pray that it serves you. You will learn and witness the five stages to achieving more freedom in your health. It will transform your life in so many ways. The five stages will take you from your state of frustration and pain to true health freedom.

No matter at what state of health you are right now, whether you are struggling with a chronic illness or looking to improve a certain area of your health, such as increasing your pace for a 5 km race, this book will help you identify, recognize, and navigate your hurdles while making positive changes for your own health and wellness.

Everything you have been through so far has brought you to this moment. I am delighted to be a part of *your* journey.

I frequently observe that once people get their health in order, they are better equipped to get other aspects of their lives in order. How you approach your health could be a reflection on how you approach other aspects of your life.

Together, let us turn your health around and get to the bottom of what is really going on with your body and your health. Let's get you going in the right direction so that *you* can get your life back.

To get well, you must change your habits and make better choices. Of course, that involves getting the right information.

I am a truth seeker, and if you are reading these words, I am confident that you are too.

Here's what you are going to learn in this book:

1. You will learn about my journey as a doctor and about my own personal health challenges, including how I overcame them.
2. You will learn about the five stages to achieving more freedom in your health and your life from frustration to freedom.
3. You will learn some tools and strategies that will empower you to get your health on the right track.

CHAPTER 1

A Picture of Health

Health is a relationship between you and your body.
~Terri Guillemets

Many of us strive to be healthy, but do we clearly understand what being healthy means?

Health can mean different things to different people and associations. Before you can comprehend where your journey will lead you, you must first understand what health is.

Before we go into the definitions, just take a moment to share your current definition of health.

My definition of health is:

____

____

____

____

____

Review your definition. Did your definition focus on symptoms or general well-being? Did you focus on what you can or can't do? Did you include lifestyle choices, or was your definition based on the amount of medications or supplements you are taking?

Compare your definition with the following definition. According to the World Health Organization, an agency of the United Nations that is concerned with international public health, "Health is a state of complete physical, mental and social well-being and not merely the absence of disease or infirmity."[2]

Did this definition mention that health is a state of being *symptom free*? No, but unfortunately, that is how many of us see it.

Health is not being symptom free. You cannot determine your health by the symptoms you have. True health is getting to the *underlying cause* of your headache or any other condition, whether it is food allergies, dehydration, toxicity, malnutrition, or lack of sleep; you need to uncover the imbalance and correct it. Healing occurs when you remove the barriers. Symptoms are only the result of your body's inability to function properly.

Here's a common scenario: You get a headache (symptom), take an ibuprofen, and the headache goes away. The ibuprofen wears off, the headache returns, you take another pill, and the cycle repeats over and over again. Is that health? Absolutely not. This is purely symptom suppression.

---

[2] "WHO Definition of Health," World Health Organization, last modified 1948, http://www.who.int/about/definition/en/print.html.

You can even be unhealthy and have no apparent symptoms.

In fact, the World Health Organization states, "Often, there are no symptoms of the underlying disease of the blood vessels. A heart attack or stroke may be the first warning of underlying disease."[3]

Health is functioning at 100 percent of your body's full potential.

Symptoms can be common, but they are never normal. And if you have *any* symptoms, it means your body is not functioning correctly.

Let's look at it this way. Imagine driving your vehicle and the check-engine light comes on. Even though you notice the light, you continue to drive, because at that moment, nothing appears to be seriously wrong with your car. You think that maybe it's just a check-engine light malfunction, so you ignore it or cover it up (suppressing the symptom) and continue to drive your vehicle.

One day, on your way to work, your automobile breaks down and leaves you stranded on the side of a busy road. Your car gets towed to the nearest mechanic, and you find out that it has serious mechanical problems. He explains the problem has been going on for quite a while and that you

[3] "Cardiovascular Diseases (CVDs)," World Health Organization, last modified March 2013, http://www.who.int/mediacentre/factsheets/fs317/en/.

could have avoided it with routine maintenance. He can repair your vehicle, but it will be very costly.

You shake your head and admit that you knew you should have kept up with the car's routine maintenance and checkups (preventive care) but just didn't make the time to get them done.

You have missed time from work, *and* you have to come up with the extra money to repair your car. Unfortunately, this is how many of us approach our health. We ignore or cover up the signs and keep moving on until it's too late.

What are your symptoms? Or what is it about your health you would like to change? Take a moment to write these down.

My symptoms / health challenges I want to eliminate:

____

____

____

____

____

If you are experiencing symptoms, you must discover what triggers them by finding the causes and eliminating them as soon as possible.

A majority of the symptoms and diseases we see today stem from chronic cellular inflammation. "Inflammation of the cell membrane affects the way the cell functions, including communication with other cells, detoxification and gene expression (DNA)."[4]

Let me give you a brief overview of how the approximately fifty trillion cells that comprise the human body function. Every one of our cells has a membrane comprised of a lipid bilayer (two walls of fat), and off these walls of fat are receptors. A normally functioning cellular membrane takes in the raw materials we eat, and our bodies break them down into usable elements. These receptors are responsible for drawing into the cell our vitamins, minerals, amino acids, and hormones like insulin.

Correlating receptors draw that raw material into the cells, and energy (ATP) is created in the mitochondria. That energy is converted into hormones, messages, and antioxidants before they are sent out of the cell to other cells. In the production of energy, toxins are also produced and released from the cell.

An inflamed cell is a congested cell. When this occurs, the receptors are blunted. The proper nutrients can't get into the cell, and toxins can't get out of the cell. This causes a number of problems with cellular function, and symptoms begin to occur in the body.

The cell then has two options:

---

[4] "R4 – Reducing Cellular Inflammation: 'The Secret Killer,'" Dr. Daniel Pompa, accessed July 13, 2013, http://drpompa.com/additional-resources/health-tips/r4-reducing-cellular-inflammation-oxidative-stress-and-nitric-oxide-cycle.

1. It will mutate or adapt to the new environment of toxicity or inflammation. This mutation is also known as cancer.
2. It will die. Also referred to as cell apoptosis or premature aging.

When the cells die off at a rapid rate, the body begins to respond with conditions like headaches, brain fog, and fatigue to more serious illnesses, such as diabetes, hypertension, and other chronic symptoms and diseases that many men and women in our culture face today.

There are three major causes of cellular inflammation. The first one is excessive sugar intake. With excessive sugar intake, the insulin receptor gets overworked and eventually dies. The cell can no longer *hear* insulin. That is what type 2 diabetes is—the body's inability to *hear* insulin, not *produce* insulin. But in today's medical treatment, medications are used to beat the pancreas into producing more insulin, when the problem is in the cell. High insulin levels drive inflammation further, eventually leading to heart disease and premature aging and will further the progression of diabetes. Insulin also makes it harder to lose weight because insulin is a fat-storing hormone. So, in order to get well, this vicious cycle has to stop.

Sugar also fights with other receptors, such as the receptors that take in vitamins and minerals and, therefore, acts as an anti-nutrient. This is why sugar plays such a huge role in many of the chronic diseases we see today.

Two hundred years ago, the average American ate only 2 pounds of sugar a year. In 1970, we ate 123 pounds of sugar per year. Today, the average American consumes almost 152 pounds of sugar in one year. This is equal to 3 pounds (or 6 cups) of sugar consumed in one week![5]

The second cause of cellular inflammation is the intake of bad fats. We have become so afraid of saturated fat and cholesterol, but when we look at the research, these are the two most necessary fats to regenerate the cell membrane.[6]

Bad fats in the form of polyunsaturated fatty acid (PUFAs) damage the cells and drive inflammation and oxidative stress (production of free radicals). These fats, in the form of vegetable oils, are found in the majority of our processed foods including chips, pies, cookies, crackers, and even foods marketed as health foods.

Sugar combined with bad fats increase the LDL particles (commonly known as bad cholesterol) that drive inflammation.

The third major cause of cellular inflammation is environmental toxins. The Environmental Protection Agency defines toxin as "any chemical or mixture that may be harmful

---

[5] "How Much Sugar Do You Eat? You May Be Surprised!" NH DHHS-DPHS-Health Promotion in Motion, accessed August 2014, http://www.dhhs.nh.gov/dphs/nhp/documents/sugar.pdf.

[6] "R4 – Reducing Cellular Inflammation: "'The Secret Killer,'" Dr. Daniel Pompa, accessed July 16, 2013, http://drpompa.com/additional-resources/health-tips/r4-reducing-cellular-inflammation-oxidative-stress-and-nitric-oxide-cycle.

to the environment and to human health if inhaled, swallowed, or absorbed through the skin."[7] Environmental toxins involve a broad entity of chemicals that we encounter in our everyday lives. Our environment has been bombarded with over 84,000 chemicals since World War II, with about 1,500 new chemicals being introduced into our air, food, and water each year.[8] Every time we take a shower, we breathe in more chlorine than is in a glass of unfiltered water. The International Agency for Research on Cancer and the World Health Organization have concluded that 80 percent of all cancers are attributed to environmental rather than genetic factors, including exposure to carcinogenic chemicals, such as formaldehyde and benzene, many of which are found in household cleaning products. Our laundry detergents, kitchen cleaners, and air fresheners could be unknowingly making us sick. Every morning we lather up in skin-care products that are also loaded with toxic chemicals, such as sodium lauryl sulfate, which has devastating effects on our health. Other toxic chemicals we have daily exposure to include fluoride, molds, pesticides, herbicides, and heavy metals like lead and mercury.

Toxins are known as the smoking gun that can trigger numerous chronic diseases, including cancer, diabetes, and obesity. The inability to lose weight, despite diet and exercise, is usually associated with high toxicity levels in the body.

---

[7] "What Is A Toxic Substance?" Environmental Protection Agency, last modified May 9, 2012, http://www.epa.gov/kidshometour/toxic.htm.

[8] "TSCA Chemical Substance Inventory," Environmental Protection Agency, last modified March 13, 2014, http://www.epa.gov/oppt/existingchemicals/pubs/tscainventory/basic.html.

Another cause of cellular inflammation I would like to introduce has helped me "crack the code" with not only my health challenges but also some of the tough cases that I've seen in my practice. I will call this the fourth cause of cellular inflammation, which is a negative belief system. Our cells not only adversely respond to a toxic or unbalanced physical environment, but they also respond to unhealthy or unsupportive beliefs.[9]

Whatever program you use or lifestyle changes you choose to implement, what you believe plays a major role in whether or not the system will work for you. Your outer world, including your health, is a reflection of your inner thoughts. When I was able to grasp this concept, I began to notice my life and the lives of others completely transform.

If you have had enough of living with the pain, discomfort, and inconvenience of what health problems can cause, then this book will help you find that missing link that may be preventing you from getting well. Even if you haven't yet been through the ringer with doctors; haven't been diagnosed with a chronic, debilitating disease; or are looking to improve your current state of health, you will also benefit from reading this book.

We are all on our own journeys. Some of us are moving more toward sickness and disease, while some of us are on the path to better health and healing. Are the choices you're making today bringing you closer to your health care goals? Or are they making you unhealthier?

---

[9] Bruce H. Lipton, PhD, *The Biology of Belief: Unleashing the Power of Consciousness, Matter & Miracles,* (Hay House, 2005), 107-114.

CHAPTER 2

My Journey

Tell your heart that the fear of suffering is worse than suffering itself. And no heart has ever suffered when it goes in search of its dream.
~ Paulo Coelho

I grew up as a "military brat." My father was in the Air Force, and we moved around quite a bit during my childhood. It had its advantages and disadvantages, but the experience exposed me to so many people and places and has played a big role in the person I am today.

My mother did her best to keep her family healthy. Her attempts to feed her kids healthy foods (or what she believed to be healthy at that time) competed with my dad's Little Debbie® snack cakes and other treats he would bring home every day after work. So you can say I had the best of both worlds … well, sort of.

I had my share of soft drinks, candy, and ice cream in my lifetime. In my invincible, young adult years, I indulged in pizza and beer with my buddies and had bread at every meal, being unaware of the impact it would have on my health in the future. I had extreme sugar cravings, especially a few days before my menstrual cycle. My favorite premenstrual snack was a Dr. Pepper® and pack of Peanut M&M's®. I also dealt with crippling menstrual cramps, severe mood swings, depression, and unattractive skin rashes. At the time, I accepted these as normal symptoms and wasn't aware that I was setting myself up for a plethora of symptoms that began to develop in my late thirties.

When I was thirteen, my father was diagnosed with type 2 diabetes. And as I grew up, I noticed that just about everyone in my family eventually received a diagnosis of this debilitating disease. It almost seemed as though everyone was just waiting on his or her turn to get it.

Many of the women in my family started small, but by the time they finished high school, they were pleasantly plump, which then turned into obesity after marriage or having children.

I was expected to gain weight after high school. It didn't happen. Then college … not too much. Then, I was supposed to gain weight after getting married and having children. This obsession was so bad I didn't want to get married and have children. However, I did get married, I did have children, and I did eventually gain the weight.

In my midtwenties, I began to notice more changes in my body. I started to experience chronic constipation and fat around my abdomen. My menstrual cramping progressively got worse, where I was literally bedridden with headaches, nausea, and vomiting. I also started to develop severe monthly urinary tract and yeast infections. I also tired easily after cardiovascular activities, such as running, going upstairs, or dancing. Doctors had prescribed pain-killers and antibiotics that only provided temporary relief. Frustrated, I began to take matters in my own hands and reduced calories or skipped meals in order to lose the extra fat. I relied on laxatives to relieve the constipation. I also began to experiment with over-the-counter appetite suppressants and energy drinks.

At age twenty-five, I had a urinary tract infection (UTI) so severe that I was unable to function. The antibiotics were ineffective, and a friend referred me to an herbalist. He educated me on a proper diet and told me to reduce my sugar intake, which was feeding the bacteria causing the infection. He recommended a protocol, including various herbs to help beat the infection. I do not remember the specifics, but I do remember that when I started the protocol, my symptoms got worse. He told me it was a normal healing reaction, because the body was finally eliminating the bacteria from my body. The medications I had taken for years only suppressed my symptoms but never completely alleviated the problem. His protocol was cleansing the bacteria from my body. I toughed it out for several days until it finally healed. I haven't had a UTI since. That experience got my attention, and I started taking basic nutrition and herbal workshops at his center.

Not too long after that, I was involved in an auto accident and suffered from severe whiplash. Pain pills and muscle relaxers only provided temporary relief. For months afterward, I was still in pain and quickly losing normal range of motion in my neck. Another friend recommended that I go see a chiropractor. I had never heard of chiropractic, but at that point, I was ready to try anything. I followed my treatment plan that included regular adjustments several times a week. The results were amazing. Within weeks, I noticed increased motion in my neck and less pain. I became more fascinated about natural healing and attended his workshops to learn more about how chiropractic worked.

With my new nutritional and herbal knowledge and regular chiropractic adjustments, I was captivated with this new way of healing. Shortly thereafter, I started teaching fitness classes, became a vegetarian, and stopped all over-the-counter and prescription drugs.

I was determined to change the direction of my health and my life. In 1998, I resigned from my position of four years as an engineer at Ford Motor Company in Dearborn, Michigan; packed my bags; and moved to Atlanta, Georgia, to pursue my chiropractic degree.

While in the demanding program, I did take time out to enjoy hiking up Kennesaw Mountain, running 5- and 10-km races, and continuing my vegetarian lifestyle. Up until that point, I thought I had been taking great care of myself. I got regular chiropractic adjustments; ate a great amount of healthy, organic food; used non-toxic skin care products; made my own bread; rarely ate fast food; and hadn't had a soft drink in years. However, I still dealt with menstrual cramping, low energy, and skin problems.

During my eight years as a vegetarian, I had consumed a diet extremely high in carbs and sugars. I now realize how this diet may have eventually put my pancreas through the stress that had set me up for the prediabetic I had eventually become. My genetic code and biggest fear had activated, and it became my mission to discover how to turn it off.

Before I had children, medical literature and their charts considered my weight to be healthy at 145 pounds for my five-foot-nine frame. But after knowing what I know today, I now realize that even though the experts considered my weight healthy, I was skinny fat and far from being healthy.

I managed to fulfill my "destiny" after the birth of my two boys. I thought I was doing the right things, and I still managed to gain over seventy pounds. Everyone was telling me it was normal, and I tried hard to believe the excuses I was hearing: "You are over thirty-five; you're supposed to gain weight!" "You're nursing; it will come off!" "Give it time!" Of course, I tried to justify it with the fact I was thirty-six and forty when I had my children, but something still felt "off," and those excuses didn't work for me.

On my forty-first birthday, July 22, 2012, I looked in the mirror and thought *enough is enough*! I weighed in at 205 pounds and barely recognized myself. My second born, was turning one in August. I had managed to lose only twenty pounds within six months after he was born, but I was struggling to shed the other fifty pounds, no matter what I did. I was doing Zumba®, weightlifting, and Pilates—the weight just wouldn't budge.

I didn't know what weight trouble was until that moment. For a natural health care practitioner who wanted to help others get healthier naturally, I couldn't get my own health in order. It was frustrating. I was ashamed and embarrassed. I was also personally dealing with headaches, fatigue, depression, lower back pain, and mood swings, not to mention fear, low self-confidence, and shame. "It's just hormones," everyone would tell me. I didn't want to hear that.

What was going on? I am a doctor! I am supposed to figure out this stuff. People relied on *me* to help *them* overcome *their* list of health issues. My biggest confession: deep down inside, I felt insecure, because I was unable to help myself. Yes, I admit, I was embarrassed and ashamed and began to doubt myself as a doctor.

In October of 2011, I was denied life insurance. I requested my lab report, and this is what I discovered:

Test	**Result**	**Normal Ranges**
GGT	174	<65 U/L
AST	72	0 – 45 U/L
ALT	127	0 – 45 U/L
Hemoglobin A1C	6.1	3.0 – 6.0%
Triglycerides	206	<150 mg/dL
Alk. Phos.	153	30 – 125 U/L
Cholesterol	276	140 – 230 mg/dL
HDL	85	35 – 55 mg/dL
LDL	149	0 – 129 mg/dL

(Go to Appendix A for a brief description of blood chemistry markers.)

They based their decision on my abnormal AST, ALT, and GGT results, which revealed my potential for severe liver and gallbladder disease. I was shocked. But I concluded that my readings were abnormal because of having a baby only two months prior to taking this test. So, we did it again in July 2012, and once again, I was denied. Here are my scores:

Test	**Result**	**Normal Ranges**
GGT	92	<65 U/L
AST	27	0 – 45 U/L
ALT	41	0 – 45 U/L
Hemoglobin A1C	5.9	3.0 – 6.0%
Triglycerides	67	<150 mg/dL
Alk. Phos.	113	30 – 125 U/L
Cholesterol	278	140 – 230 mg/dL
HDL	99	35 – 55 mg/dL
LDL	166	0 – 129 mg/dL

There was some improvement, but cholesterol was still high, my hemoglobin A1C indicated I was prediabetic, and my elevated gamma-glutamyl transpeptidase (GGT) suggested possible bile duct or liver disease. Elevated levels are also found in heavy drinkers. So of course, the life insurance inquired about my drinking history. They were concerned about whether or not I was an alcoholic. They asked me if I had been to any AA meetings and other probing questions about my drinking history. I was offended. I did have more than enough cheap beer, wine, and liquor on the weekends in college. But after a pretty bad hangover, I decided it was time to slow down, and it became more casual and social. I stopped drinking completely in 2007 when I learned I was pregnant with my first child.

After my pity party, I began my mission to find answers. Due to frustration, I came to the point that I had to heal my body not just for my sake but also for my children's sake. I knew that if I didn't get this under control now, I was likely to lose my gallbladder or develop heart disease or diabetes, just like many others in my family had. I've seen what it can do to the body, and I didn't want it to happen to me.

This was a major turning point in my health, my future, and the way I run my practice. This part of my journey has made me a better mother, wife, and practitioner.

Once I decided to change my circumstances, I began to notice opportunities that guided me on my journey. I noticed an online advertisement for a Health Center of the Future (HCF) seminar lead by Dr. Daniel Pompa.[10] It was a nutrition seminar, and at the time, I thought I already knew what I had to know. I had already had extensive training in nutrition and functional medicine, so I just hit the delete button. *That's what the ego will do to you.*

For months, I kept getting e-mails to join their mailing list for online videos, and it was some time after my second set of

---

[10] HCF Seminars, http://www.hcfseminars.com.

blood tests when I was more open to look into it. So, I entered my contact information. I didn't watch the videos right away, but I did get a personal phone call inviting me to their next seminar in Las Vegas in November. I was still nursing at the time, and I wasn't ready to leave my baby for an extended period of time. Because of my circumstances, I elected to do the live-stream broadcast and was able to watch the event from the comfort of my own home. I must say, I had my eyes glued to my laptop the whole weekend.

This was the first time I had learned of cellular healing. Dr. Pompa and other speakers discussed the causes of cellular inflammation, and I immediately applied The Cellular Healing Diet[11]. I increased my fat intake and stopped eating inflammatory foods, such as grains and sugars. To get healthy, you heal and regenerate at the cellular level.

Then there was a segment with Jordan Rubin, the founder of Garden of Life[12] and Beyond Organic[13], who shared his journey of personal health challenges with severe life-threatening, gastrointestinal problems. He explained how he overcame them by introducing healing foods into his diet.

Looking back, I had a strong addiction to bread. Yes, the quality had evolved from store-bought, whole wheat bread to homemade bread, but it was still an issue and was one of my triggers to becoming weight-loss resistant. And if it

---

[11] The Cellular Healing Diet, http://www.CellularHealingDiet.com.

[12] Garden of Life, http://www.GardenofLife.com.

[13] Beyond Organic, http://DrLeona.MyBeyondOrganic.com.

wasn't bread, it was potato or corn chips. These foods are not included in The Cellular Healing Diet.

I was intrigued. I read *Wheat Belly*[14] by William Davis, MD and many other books on this topic. The course of my nutrition and wellness programs began to change for the better. I took all my patients off grains. I started to experiment with grain-free recipes. I kept studying, I incorporated new food guidelines in my life, and I was discovering how to heal my body at the cellular level. By May of 2013 (six months), I had lost another twenty pounds. My depression decreased, my headaches were gone, and I was starting to see some significant improvement in my blood work.

Don't get me wrong. There were some weeks when I didn't lose weight and felt discouraged. But what picked me back up were my support groups and my reasons for starting in the first place. What I desired became bigger than the challenges. That's when it started to click. Many gave up, including my own patients, because their expectations weren't being met, they didn't believe in their bodies' true innate ability to heal, or they didn't have the right support system. This experience taught me that in order to see the results, I had to trust and be patient with the healing process. I stopped believing in the illness and began believing in the healing.

This became more than just looking good in clothes. This evolved more into changing my inner world. Once I changed my mind-set, I began to deal with my fears, doubts,

---

[14] William Davis, MD. *Wheat Belly: Lose the Wheat, Lose the Weight, and Find Your Path Back to Health,* (Rodale Books, 2011).

and disbeliefs that were holding me back. I noticed how my health was directly proportional to my state of mind. It was about me ensuring I took steps in the direction that would bring me closer to health and wellness and away from sickness and disease. It was about establishing the right patterns and creating new, healthier habits. It was about becoming happier, becoming confident, and being able to love myself and embrace the life that I had and those in it.

At the writing of this book, I am 160 pounds. I have gone from a size 22 to a size 10. I am still working on other aspects of my health, such as building more muscle mass and improving endurance. I continue to enjoy distance running, Zumba®, and CrossFit. At forty-three years old, I feel better and have more energy than ever! I maintain what I have achieved by incorporating a lifestyle that includes The Cellular Healing Diet, fasting, and cellular detox. I continue to learn and study programs that address the barriers to healing and the connections of how our beliefs affect our health.

CHAPTER 3

The Five Stages to Freedom

Healing is a matter of time, but it is sometimes also a matter of opportunity.

~Hippocrates

The journey to healing can be broken down into five stages. These stages came together as I studied other avenues of health, spirituality, and self-improvement. I have learned from well-known experts, read books, and taken extensive courses on topics such as healing techniques, obtaining financial freedom, managing business, and finding true purpose in life. These stages can be applied to other aspirations, such as building a successful business or getting a better handle on finances.

In my early days of practice, patients wouldn't commit to care. I assumed that they were the problem, they didn't understand or appreciate the work I did, or they didn't find their health to be a priority. As time went on, I discovered that it was not the patients who were the problem. It was me.

My client base could only grow as much as I could. As I began to work on my inner world, my outer world and my ability to help others expanded. I had to learn to manage my time, my finances, and my body before I could expect it of others. Once I got that, everything else fell into place. Better health provided more clarity in what I needed to do, more energy to get it done, and more passion to share it with others. I had to stop looking for the magic bullet that would help me reach more clients. What I had to do was work on me. In my search, I began to identify the following five stages that all successful people go through. You will recognize them in your journey, and understanding each phase empowers you to stay on track and move forward.

Stage One: Frustration

You are tired of living with symptoms. You are frustrated with doing things that don't work or make you feel worse. You are looking for real answers and real results. You are ready for a change and ready to get well and stay well.

This is the stage where you begin to search for answers. You may find yourself constantly stuck in this stage, or you may find yourself here over and over again despite what you do. Whatever the case, you are at a point of frustration and being overwhelmed, and you are ready for change.

It is this *pain* that drives you to change. This source of pain is your *why*. For most of us, in order to make big changes in our lives, we need a strong and compelling why. Typically, the more intense the pain and suffering, the stronger the desire to change.

Here are some examples that may drive you to change:

- Chronic depression or lack of enthusiasm about life
- Lack of energy and stamina to take care of yourself or your children
- Fear of being a burden on family members
- Loss of a loved one to a debilitating disease
- Severe or life-threatening diagnosis

The impact is different for everybody and at different times. But at stage one, you have reached a tipping point and you are ready to do something different.

For example, you look in the mirror one day and you don't like what you see. You notice extra fat around the hips, waist, and thighs. Your clothes don't fit right, and you are starting to feel insecure about your body. You don't go out with your friends because you don't want other people to see you this way.

The bad news is that too many of us do not even go beyond this stage. I don't doubt that we all desire to have more, do more, or be more, but we continue to dwell at this stage. Why? It's usually because of fear, doubt, and disbelief. We may have failed in the past, our expectations weren't met, or we have given up too soon. Possibly, we are just afraid of what we may have to give up in the process, or we simply are afraid to step out of our comfort zones.

Not only is fear of failure a factor but also the fear of success. Concerns about what our friends or spouses will think of us or whether or not they will accept the changes we plan to make can lock us into this stage.

If you want better health bad enough, you will focus more on the reasons that a healthy lifestyle will bring. Expecting the worst will not get you closer to progress.

If you are not at the point of frustration yet or don't feel motivated to change, that's okay. You will know when you are ready. Be patient with the process. Life has a way of tipping the scales until we are compelled to act in harmony with our environments and ourselves. We cannot force ourselves to do something we are not ready to do. Be present. Look at your current circumstances. What are you ready to change? What are you concerned about? What are you telling yourself?

Stage Two: Faith

You believe you can achieve what you set out to do. You begin to envision the end from the beginning. You begin to think about all the things you will be able to do—how you will look and feel and how your life will change. You have found hope.

At stage two, you begin to feel positive about your future again, and you envision yourself thinner, feeling younger, having more energy, traveling with your family, and so on. You now realize that you co-create your life. Better health is your choice. You acknowledge your situations, and you believe you can overcome them. You begin to believe and trust in the process.

In the faith stage, you are constantly visualizing what you would like to become or restore, even though you are not yet quite sure how you will get there. Nonetheless, your confidence is extremely strong at this stage.

You may have found yourself in a situation where you have been stuck between stages one and two because you don't believe you deserve it. Back to our example, you look in the mirror again. You imagine a smaller waistline and firmer thighs and hips. You pull out an old pair of your favorite jeans and see yourself comfortably in them. You see yourself smiling and more confident. You know it is now up to you to make this a reality.

Stage Three: Firm Commitment

When you are committed to getting well, lifestyle changes are required; it takes new habits in order to get new results. They require time and consistency.

Stage three is where all the work begins. Goals and an action plan have been set. You have an idea of what direction you need to take. You have a plan, and you have made a firm commitment to start taking action.

To change your health, you begin to learn how to live differently. Several things in your normal routine begin to change. You may have to wake up earlier to fit in your new exercise routine. There are things you must omit from your diet or lifestyle. You may have to learn to prepare your meals at home, instead of going to a drive through every night. You learn that you have to make special accommodations for travel or special outings. Many of the new things you learn may be confusing or challenging, but at this stage, you give it your best effort because you want to feel better.

Unfortunately, because of the new habits and work that is involved, I estimate that 50 percent begin to back out at this stage. It is at this stage where a strong why provides you the strength to get through it. When it gets tough, you must hold on to why you started in the first place. When your why and your commitment are strong, you won't let little distractions or excuses get in the way. You will stick to your commitment long enough to see some amazing results. Of course, you must also maintain a strong conviction throughout the process.

Committed to losing fifteen pounds by summer, you get a membership at the new gym up the street. You also hire a trainer and sign up for a six-month training program, complete with diet recommendations and an exercise plan to help meet your goals. You commit to completing the program no matter what.

Implementation and consistency are required during this stage if you want to see results. Sometimes it will be hard and challenging; sometimes it will be fun and easy. Just trust the process.

Stage Four: Feeling Discouraged

You have begun to take action, but you are not getting the results you expected or you've hit a plateau. You begin to realize it is not as easy as you had hoped it would be. You become impatient; you contemplate quitting.

It is realistic to believe that 99 percent of people tend to turn back at this stage.

Getting healthier at first seems easy, but it is not simple. You are going to have good days and bad days. You are going to have successes and failures. Whenever you get stuck, it means it is time to reassess your situation and make the necessary adjustments. Some people fail to go beyond stage four because they get tired of waiting or the program doesn't meet their expectations. As a result, they end right back at stage one, frustrated, believing that what they were doing was not working.

I find that at this stage, you learn the most about yourself and learn what you are capable of achieving. You face certain fears, challenges, and limited beliefs about yourself. Until you face them, you are more likely to repeat the same patterns over and over again.

Don't let discouragement get the best of you and persuade you to give up. Overcoming the obstacles is what makes you more resilient and confident.

If you have been working out regularly for two months but are discouraged because you haven't been losing weight as quickly as you would have liked, this is the stage where you need to reassess your plan and adjust it as necessary. Do you need to work out at a different time? Are you eating too many carbohydrates? Do you need to change the type of exercise you are doing? Are you sabotaging your efforts?

Remember, you didn't get overweight or sick overnight, so you can't expect to get well overnight. Keep patient and keep moving forward.

At this stage, it is also crucial you get the right support. I tell my patients that when things get rough, schedule time to speak to me so that we can get them over their hurdles. I can't say enough about how important a support system is when you are making some big changes in your life.

The sad truth about this is, in many cases, when you feel impatient and ready to quit, you may be closer than you think to your breakthrough. You may not ever get to experience freedom because you gave up too soon.

Stage Five: Freedom

You have had a breakthrough. You are starting to see amazing results. You are a different person. You are more inspired to stay on track and encourage others to do the same.

You may have heard or know of someone who has made a miraculous healing recovery. There are so many stories of people who have recovered from life-threatening diseases, such as cancer or a serious brain injury. But it doesn't have to be that drastic. It could be better athletic performance, a ten- to fifteen-pound weight loss, or a good night's rest.

What matters at this stage is that you are experiencing change. Your pain doesn't wake you up at night. You notice more energy, or you are able to decrease the amount of medications you are taking. You have fallen down only to get right back up. You are stronger, more confident. You are getting closer to the bigger picture of whatever it is that you wanted to accomplish, and you keep moving forward until you get there. With faith, patience, and commitment, you are beginning to get your life back, and you are inspired to help others do the same. This is freedom! This is what we strive for. But before you get to this point, you have to survive through the other stages. You have to get through the tough days and appreciate the great ones.

CHAPTER 4

Stage One: Frustration

It's pain that changes our lives.
~ Steve Martin

It's Monday, 7:00 a.m. I roll over to hit the snooze button and then, drudgingly, roll over on my back and stare at the ceiling. I curse to myself because it's another morning, and my exhausting, weekly routine begins all over again.

I know I should be thankful for my family, my home, and my career, but I struggle with this constant fatigue and depression and tend to drag throughout the day. My zest and excitement for life is simply ... gone. I am not ready to get out of this bed and start my day. It doesn't help that I tossed and turned all night long. I would give anything for a good night's rest.

Beep, beep, beep. There goes the alarm *again*. Reluctantly, I drag myself out of the bed and find my way through the dimly lit room to the bathroom. And just like I do every morning, I use the bathroom, brush my teeth, and then jump in the shower. As I dry off, I catch a glimpse of myself in the foggy mirror. I am so disgusted with myself. I have a double chin, an ugly roll of fat around my waistline *and* on my back, and the most unattractive dents on my thighs. Then I aversely jump on the scale—205 pounds! How did I let myself get this way?

I have been running my own wellness practice for six years and still struggling to make ends meet. I am up to my eyeballs in debt, patients don't seem to want what I have to offer, patients aren't showing up for their appointments, checks are bouncing, and I am always sending someone to collections.

Some patients got well quickly, some slowly; some didn't appear to be getting well at all. Some followed my recommendations; some didn't. Some blamed me for everything that went wrong in their lives.

This stress led me to hire practice-management coaches and read self-improvement books, searching for the answers to my failures. I frequently went to chiropractic technique, functional medicine and nutrition seminars, searching for the solutions that would help me get my patients well. I applied what I learned to my own body as well. I frequently introduced new techniques or products and still lacked improvement I was looking for. I tried different marketing methods to attract more potential clients. They would come in and not go beyond the first visit. I was beginning to doubt my skills as a doctor and rethink my path.

I started to compare myself with colleagues who had graduated around the same time I had and appeared to me more successful. Why was I struggling? I was putting in the long hours. I had the knowledge. What was I doing wrong? Why wasn't my practice growing? These trials were taking a toll on me mentally and physically.

The effort I was putting into growing my practice was causing my health to slowly deteriorate. My energy was plummeting. I fought to get through each day. I wanted to quit every other weekend. I was worried about my future and my position I had taken on as a doctor.

The struggle amplified after I had my first son in 2008. New challenges came into the mix. I had lost six cups of blood during the birth. My fatigue, headaches, and depression had gotten worse. He was a fussy baby, and I got even less sleep at night. I wasn't in the position to take much time off. The office had been closed for two weeks, the bills were piling up, and against my midwife's wishes, I returned to work after two weeks. I started back at two to three half days per week. I was nursing, and I felt it best to bring my baby to the office with me.

Having my baby with me turned the dynamics around in my office. I even had patients walk away because I had my baby in the office. He cried frequently and would only stop in the comfort of my arms. My professionalism was being questioned, but in my heart, it felt like the right thing to do for him at the time. I was a mother and a doctor, and I was trying to juggle both. It wasn't fair to my patients to be distracted by my personal life. It is hard to be there for your patients when you are worried about your crying child or if you are going to make your mortgage payment. I worked hard to keep up appearances that everything was all right. Deep down inside, I was extremely worried about what my patients thought. I was exhausted with this battle and was ready to quit. I cried frequently. Somehow, I found the strength to keep moving on.

I began to have dreams of being homeless on the street with my baby. Fear was setting in, and I started to experience anxiety. What will happen if my career doesn't work out? What will happen if I cannot provide for my family? This financial burden created stress in my marriage. My husband's income at the time was not enough to handle the massive debt I had accumulated. I managed to make ends meet for several more years. Literally, with my child on my back, I kept treating the patients. But I was still unhappy, tired of struggling and wondering if I should be doing something else with my life.

I signed up for more seminars, hoping to find the missing ingredient that was preventing me from achieving the practice of my dreams and helping more people. I incorporated more nutrition and lifestyle programs in my office.

By 2011 three more years of a roller coaster practice had passed, and I was expecting my second child. During my second pregnancy, I dealt with gestational diabetes. I will never forget how I just broke down and cried after learning my fetus was at risk if I didn't get my sugar levels under control. The problem didn't go away after he was born. My sugar levels still had to be tightly controlled or I would be at risk of getting type 2 diabetes.

This time I had gotten some help in the office. I was sharing my office space with another chiropractor. She treated my patients while I was on maternity leave. Instead of taking two weeks off, I took off two months. Dynamics changed again, and I was taking care of two boys instead of one. I brought my second baby to the office just like I had the first one. He was a lot quieter, though, and patients didn't even notice he was there. At some levels, I was doing better in practice; it was my health that was preventing me from doing what needed to be done. I had gained seventy pounds since beginning private practice and birthing my children. My physical appearance began to affect me mentally. I didn't exercise as much as I used to before I had children. I started running again but still struggled with getting my body to bounce back.

My self-confidence was shattered. I got tired of people who were amazed at how well I ate and still had weight issues. They weren't aware I had prediabetes, fatty liver, and a congested gall bladder. I was also dealing with constipation and bloating, and the list kept getting longer and longer. I added another supplement, did another cleanse, ran more frequently, but I still wasn't feeling better.

How would people listen to me when I didn't look like the picture of health? I leaned on the excuse that I had just had a baby, but that excuse got weaker as the baby got older. I had convinced myself that I was a failure.

I got the homeless dream again, and it seemed more dramatic, more real. It caused me to sit upright, sweating, with my heart beating out of my chest. Then the question came up. What would happen to my children if something happened to me? I was at risk for diabetes and heart disease. I didn't want to go down that road. Enough was enough. I was tired of feeling sorry for myself, was ready to take another path, and wanted to help others do the same. I was ready to change.

My story is not unique. Like many women, I was really struggling to get through the day and take care of my family. Despite the research and the many efforts to do and feel better, I still suffered from headaches, fatigue, depression, and weight gain, with more and more symptoms adding to my list.

This is a tough stage because questions, pain, anxiety, and feeling overwhelmed dwell here. We start to ask ourselves, *why is this happening to me? What am I doing wrong?* We may begin to isolate ourselves and feel that no one understands what we are going through. Fear may consume us and prevent us from taking action.

Then there is the tendency to take care of others at the expense of ourselves. Oftentimes, we do so much for our family members, coworkers, friends, and even patients that we fail to put our personal health as a top priority.

The truth is that those who depend on us will also start to suffer, because as the decline of our health starts to affect our daily tasks, we become less effective and less available. Our loved ones will begin to feel the effects of our deteriorating health, if they haven't already.

We have to fight against the negative self-chatter that goes on and on in our heads, such as *I can't do this* or *I don't deserve this*. These incessant thoughts are common—often far more common than we know. These thoughts can bind our physical and emotional ability to push out of the frustration stage.

Journey Notes:

Now, let's take a moment to reflect on where you are and what you would like to change in regard to your health. Sometimes we get so wrapped up in the stress and hustle and bustle of our everyday lives, we don't take the time to see where we are right now. It is these quiet, still moments that direct us. We have to stop every now and then to see where to go or what to do next. At the end of each stage, there will be the opportunity to reflect and direct the process of your journey.

You can begin to turn this cycle around by knowing that you can come out of this stage realizing:

You are vital to the longevity of your life.

Your effectiveness largely depends on your mental and physical strength.

You cannot keep promises when you are operating on empty.

Answer the following questions:

On a scale of one to ten, how would you rate your general health? (One being chronically ill and ten being extremely healthy.)

What concerns you the most about your health?

How long have you been dealing with the above condition(s)?

What is your day like when your health is at its worse?

Why do you want to change it?

What do you believe has contributed to your current state of health?

What do you believe has prevented you from improving your health?

Do you believe *you* can change the course of your health?

Are you ready to get rid of this problem(s)?

CHAPTER 5

Stage Two: Faith

At the end of the day, we must go forward with hope and not backward by fear and division.
~ Jesse Jackson

Not only was I frustrated with my health, but I also didn't feel competent enough to help others. I hate to make that confession, but it's true. Not only was my health at stake, but I also felt responsible for the role I played in my community to help others get well. I could not lead people to places I had not been, and it was time to change my course of action.

Everything I did was holistic, and I didn't have to resort to any medications or surgery, which I wanted to avoid at all costs. I was aware of the risks and side effects, and changing my lifestyle and getting to the root cause was my focus. Commonly, muscle relaxers are prescribed for pain and antidepressants for depression and mood swings. Medications suppress the symptoms and only provide a temporary fix.

They do not address the underlying cause. The body does the healing if we remove the barriers.

Frustrated with my current circumstances, I was ready to keep searching for the missing piece of the puzzle. I kept reading, kept attending seminars, and kept picking the brains of successful healthcare practitioners. Because of my new intention to get out of the situation I was in, I began to see things with new eyes. I had the tools; when I changed my mind, things began to happen. Instead of focusing on how overwhelmed I was with running a practice, taking care of my family, and taking care of me, I focused on the possibility of healing and how my life could change.

In one of the HCF seminars I attended, we had learned to do a visualization exercise. We had to close our eyes and imagine our futures. First, we had to imagine what our lives would be like if we didn't change. I went five years out and imagined living with heart disease; complications of type 2 diabetes; and not being able to chase after my boys, attend their sporting events, or go camping with them. That was not the road I wanted to take.

If I kept doing the same thing over and over, I would only bring more frustration in my life. This cycle is what greatly contributed to my depression. The stress also contributed to more weight gain, more fatigue, and more desperation.

Then we had to visualize the lives that we could have if we took the right action. I began focusing on fitting back into my size ten jeans and being able to hike, dance, and run up the stairs without losing my breath. I envisioned having an abundance of energy to spend quality time with my boys. I imagined myself kicking a ball with them in the front yard or chasing them at the beach. I saw my practice growing, helping others overcome health challenges. I saw myself as more of a leader, advisor, and teacher. As a doctor, I do not do the healing; I assist in the healing process. I had systems in place that educated and inspired; my profession became more of a mission and less of a job. It was more than dispensing another supplement or providing another chiropractic adjustment; it was about transforming lives.

As I was doing this visualization exercise, I realized I did have the knowledge and the skills to succeed. The problem was I was so busy thinking about how bad things were that I couldn't allow the good things to happen. My inner world or my mind-set was not congruent with my actions. I was unable to bring more of what I did want because I focused too much on what I didn't want.

What you focus on expands. If you focus on your fatigue, you will get more fatigue. If you focus on your belly fat, you will get more belly fat. Worrying about your high blood pressure will raise your blood pressure. Acknowledge where you are today, but understand that you don't have to stay there. Be clear on what you want. Believe that it is real. Your actions will follow your solid vision. Allow flexibility. Your desires may change, and that is okay. That is the most interesting part of the journey.

It's fun to visualize. These mental pictures can inspire you. To keep these visions at the top of my mind, I post pictures of a fit body or motivational quotes around my house and office. I listen to audio, I read books, and I attend live events. I feed my mind with what I desire. I study what other successful people do. Before you can achieve it, you have to see it, feel it, and completely believe it. Immerse yourself in it, and monitor those negative pictures. When they pop up, replace them with a positive thought. Stop dwelling in the past and giving the illness all the attention. Trust and have faith in your healing.

At stage two, it is important to note that once you enter it, there are some surefire ways to stay focused on your vision while traveling through the rest of your journey to better health. When excitement and hope enter your emotional systems, you cannot help but feel that you can accomplish anything. It's a great feeling! It can become a reality but will require lots of work and persistence from you, especially when times get rough.

There will be times when you may want to go back to the stage of frustration. To reduce the chances of that occurring, take notes, jot down your goals, and share them with an accountability partner, such as a best friend or health coach. Make sure it is someone who is supportive and encouraging. Writing goals down is a powerful measure of your desire to complete each one, and the physical act of doing this consistently yields results sooner than you thought possible. Be free when you explore what you want. Don't be concerned about whether or not you will have it or wonder how you will get there. Be honest with yourself and clear in what you want.

One of the keys to success is to have a clear vision of what you want. For example, don't just say you want to lose weight. How much weight do you want to lose? How will you look? What kinds of clothes are you wearing? See yourself at your ideal weight. Have fun with the next exercise in discovering what you want regarding your health and your life.

Journey Notes:

Let's begin with the end in mind.

First, imagine what your life would be like one to five years from now if you did nothing to change your health.

- What is your life like?
- Are you still working?
- Do you have enough energy to take care of yourself and your family?
- How do you feel? Are you sad? Irritable? Uncomfortable?
- What do you see in the mirror? Do you like what you see? Look at your skin, hair, and nails. Do they look healthy?
- Are you spending quality time with friends and family?
- Are you taking medications? Recovering from surgery?

Now, picture yourself one year from now as if you have found a solution to your health problems. It is important to be specific.

- How do you feel? Do you notice more energy? Are you sleeping better? Do you feel less irritable? Feel less pain?
- How much weight have you lost?
- What does your skin look like? Is it more radiant?
- Are you more active? More productive?

Now, picture yourself five years from now as if you have found a solution to your health problems.

- What is your life like? Are you active? Are you traveling? Are you spending quality time with friends and family?
- What do you look like? Are you in shape? How do you look in your clothes? Are your hair and skin glowing?
- How do you feel? Do you feel confident? Strong? Energetic?

Hold on tightly to this vision. This is what will keep you strong during your journey.

CHAPTER 6

Stage Three: Firm Commitment

Vision without action is daydream. Action without vision is nightmare.
~ Japanese Proverb

You now have your vision of healing and gaining your life back planted firmly in your mind. You have that vision held so strongly in your belief system that you can feel it. It is important to truly believe and be clear in what you want. You must also firmly believe that you deserve to achieve it.

The bridge between making our fantasy, dream, or vision a reality is action. Your vision will inspire you to commit to a specific course of action involving consistent action steps that will help you reach your goal over time. Sometimes certain actions may seem hard or inconvenient. But as you will learn along your journey, these challenges will push and guide you into the direction you need to go.

I invested in many programs that failed to give me the results I was expecting. There are many different health systems and techniques available today, and I've learned that the problem was rarely the program. It was *me*. It was either me not following the instructions as thoroughly as possible or not sticking with a program long enough to see results. It was me not believing in the product. It was me lacking the commitment to see it through.

Once I started analyzing my limiting beliefs and came face to face with my current situation, it became easier to commit to the required action. I had realized from personal experience and from working with patients that if our mind-sets didn't consist of determination or commitment or if we didn't believe or trust in the process, we reduced our chances of getting well. Another powerful aspect of having clarity is this: when we are clear on the health or the life we want to achieve, circumstances will fall in our favor to help us achieve it. The steps no longer feel like an uphill battle. We begin to embrace the challenges instead of letting them defeat us.

The steps I recommend in this chapter revolve around removing the barriers to healing and restoring the building blocks of our bodies—the cells. I understand that when it comes to achieving better health, there are dozens of effective techniques and products available. I am familiar with many of them, and as we are all individuals, we have to choose what feels right for us. I now strongly believe that after years of personal and professional experience, no protocol, doctor, or medicine can assist in the healing process until we believe it can. So, as I share some of the action steps that have worked for me and a majority of my patients, keep an open mind in regard to my approach and other techniques you encounter. Learn to listen to your body, and allow its wisdom to guide you. We are our own best doctors, and ultimately it is up to us to direct our healing. Doctors and other health professionals should be only regarded as guides who assist and monitor the healing process.[15]

One of the action steps I recommend is keeping a daily journal, logging your food and beverages. The purpose of the journal is to become more aware of your eating habits and how your body responds to them. Too many of us are eating in automatic mode, and it becomes habitual. Some of us are not even aware of how much we are actually eating. Until you write it down, you will not be completely aware of what and how much you are putting into your mouth.

As you keep your journal, what habits do you recognize?

- Are you skipping meals?
- Do you eat on the run?
- Are you snacking late at night?

What types of food are you eating?

- Are you eating whole foods, such as fruits, vegetables, and meats, or is it primarily processed or packaged foods?
- Do you eat out or dine at home?
- How's your water intake?

[15] Barbara Dewey, *As You Believe*, (Bartholomew Books, 1985), 139.

Answer these questions as you review your diary and start to observe where you can make the most changes.

The purpose of this journal is not to make you feel bad or guilty. It's to help you recognize where you need to make changes. The last thing I want to encourage is guilt and the need to be perfect. Achieve success by making small but consistent improvements over time, and the journal is there to assist you in determining what areas you need to make those improvements.

You could also include how you feel, your sugar levels, or your blood pressure levels if needed. I have found this action to play a powerful role in the healing process.

As you continue to learn and understand your body during the journey, you will begin to create new healthier habits. Don't stress out on eliminating too many of the foods you can't have right away, without replacing them with more of the foods you can have. Most people do better with adding in more of the good foods they can have before they start eliminating what they shouldn't have.

Another important action step is performing a thorough health assessment that includes a comprehensive blood chemistry panel to measure the degree of cellular inflammation. A more comprehensive assessment is necessary, along with a thorough health history and a physical examination to provide a vivid picture of what is really going on in the body and what we can do to fix it. I have administered this type of evaluation to new patients during their initial stages of care to learn about their states of health and sources of illness. The blood chemistry analysis will identify particular imbalances and abnormalities. Very few medical doctors will order these types of tests and oftentimes will diagnose "in theory" based on the symptoms you provide them.

So why isn't more comprehensive testing done in doctors' offices? Let me put it this way. For some time now, there has been a decline in the quality of healthcare in the United States, in which profit takes priority over comprehensive health examinations. This is largely due to managed health care and HMO programs.[16] The current model used by these programs is more or less a disease-management system. Whereas, the comprehensive blood chemistry panel provides early detection and often prevention of disease and illness.

Comprehensive blood testing is considered extraneous under their guidelines and is therefore not covered. This is why the use of comprehensive blood testing is nonexistent, which oftentimes leads to overlooked and/or misdiagnosed illnesses or diseases.

Lab results establish a baseline and provide the information needed to determine the severity of your condition and some insight on the underlying cause of your health problems. They are also used as a tool to determine your degree of inflammation and assist in preparing your treatment program specifically designed for your health care needs.

Understanding what is going on in your body will outline the steps that are required to get you well.

---

[16] Merriam-Webster definition of HMO, http://www.merriam-webster.com/medical/hmo, accessed October 20, 2014.

In my case, labs revealed I was prediabetic. It was crucial that I reduce cellular inflammation by controlling my glucose and insulin levels.

My previous vegetarian diet of high-carb, high-sugar foods for eight years, even though it was primarily organic, was driving my inflammation. I am not just referring to the ice cream, cookies, and other dessert-like foods that we commonly associate with being high in sugar; I am also referring to the sugar hidden in our condiments and beverages. Even grains, such as whole wheat bread, corn, and oatmeal, contribute to this inflammatory process.

So, the intention of my action steps was to downregulate cellular inflammation, start a diet that promoted cellular healing, and remove excess toxins from my body.

To fix and detox the cells, I implemented the 5Rs of True Cellular Detox. The 5Rs act as a roadmap to regulating the cells' ability to heal and detox.

An Introduction to the 5Rs

The 5Rs of True Cellular Detox, a model developed by Dr. Daniel Pompa, is subsequently the best approach to fix the cells and improve the body's functions. Let's briefly go over the 5Rs to cellular detox.

R1: Remove the Source

Removing the source is, unfortunately, one of the most overlooked Rs. In order to control numerous serious conditions like diabetes or heart disease, it is very important to remove the source. Most of the healthcare practitioners, including allopathic and alternative, treat the symptoms of chronic illness without considering the primary cause or source. Instead of getting to the source, which may be toxic in nature, most practitioners dabble with downstream symptoms in their attempts to fix the issue.

We must remove the interference. If we don't remove the barriers to healing, the patients will not get well long-term.

R2: Regenerate the Cell Membrane

While removing toxins from the body, it is very important to regenerate the inner and outer cell membrane. If the cell membrane is inflamed, it will not allow nutrients to enter the cell and toxins to exit.

When the membrane is regenerated, it is able to communicate properly with other cells and bring changes in the DNA and in gene expression. If the cell membrane is unable to regenerate, it will not be able to detox or change gene expression.

Regenerating the cell membrane may be the most important R of all. We can't get the patient well without fixing the cell membrane.

R3: Restore Cellular Energy (ATP)

It is very important to restore cellular energy. In fact, increasing cellular energy is the first step to improving overall health. Without restoring cellular energy, it will be challenging to benefit from other treatments. The cells will not have sufficient energy to function properly.

With lower cellular energy, inflammation will increase. Due to this, you will feel very lethargic and lazy. You might not have the energy to get out of bed or even get through the day. In addition, you may experience some general pain and brain fog. This defect in basic cellular metabolism may be the primary cause of your illness. It is necessary to restore cellular energy to improve your condition.

R4: Reduce Inflammation and Oxidative Stress in the Cells

As mentioned earlier, it is extremely important to reduce inflammation to control chronic illness. With this stress, healing at the cellular level is certainly not possible. In order to reduce inflammation, it is crucial to reduce oxidative stress. If you're unable to reduce oxidative stress, your detox attempts are likely to fail. R4 is the most basic of the 5Rs, and the key treatment to reversing this is with The Cellular Healing Diet.

R5: Reestablish Methylation Pathways

Methylation is a standard process in which the body performs and manages many responsibilities. One of the most important responsibilities of this process is to turn the good genes on and bad genes off. Detoxification of bad hormones, such as toxic estrogen, which is linked to so many cancers today, is another responsibility of methylation. In fact, this process is the key to starting and stopping most cellular functions. Thus, it may be considered a process to sustain life.

Stress is one of the most important factors for depletion of methyl groups. It is important to understand that the human body considers physical, emotional, and chemical stress to be the same. Therefore, it responds in the same way to every kind of stress. Stress puts your DNA at risk.

You also need to take care of the chemical exposure from various products that may be toxic. Some of these include personal care products, nonorganic foods, silver amalgam fillings, city water, grain-fed meats, vaccinations, and so on. When you add these toxic substances with other stressors (emotional or physical), methyl depletion will cause some serious health problems.

"Fix the cell and you can get well."

– Dr. Daniel Pompa

My focus on the 5Rs has helped my patients and me recover from many chronic diseases and improve overall health. I use various combinations of the 5Rs throughout patients' treatment plans to help get their health back. With this approach, it is such a joy to see my patients feel better, lose weight, gain more energy, and transform their lives!

Using the 5Rs as a roadmap, I was able to manage my insulin/weight loss resistance by reducing cellular inflammation and restoring cellular and hormonal function. I was clear as to what I needed to do, not only for me but also for my family and for my patients. I was ready to change, I had faith that I would recover my health, and I was strongly committed to the process. It was challenging for me, at times, but I was more afraid of what would happen if I didn't step up to the plate. I chose to go in the direction that would bring me health, not more sickness.

I had to handle my health issues in stages by addressing the priority first. To reduce inflammation, I began The Cellular Healing Diet, eliminating my intake of inflammatory grains and sugars and increasing my intake of good fats that help rejuvenate the cell membranes. These changes alone helped encourage more weight loss, improve energy, and improve digestion.

It is important I explain why these changes were important, because there is so much confusion on this topic. We have been told to avoid saturated fats and cholesterol and to eat our whole grains every day. But since we have been given that advice, obesity and heart disease has become an epidemic in this country.[17]

Numerous studies have shown that total cholesterol is irrelevant when it comes to determining inflammation and risk of heart disease, but it is still a major concern for many people.[18]

Cholesterol is our friend. Every cell in the body needs it. Cholesterol works on the membranes so neurotransmitters can work. That is why people with low cholesterol tend to suffer from depression. Deficiencies in cholesterol can also cause violent behavior, cancer, and low libido and can make people more susceptible to strokes. Cholesterol plays a critical role in cell-to-cell communication as well as makes hormones. Cholesterol acts as an antioxidant, prevents cancer, and protects cell membranes. Our friendly cholesterol also protects our skin from sun damage, fights infections, and supports glucose metabolism.

In a health analysis, it's not the total cholesterol that matters. What matters are the number and size of the particles that carry the cholesterol.

To simplify things, I will use an analogy. In this analogy, think of a car as the LDL particle and the people inside the

---

[17] Lee S. Gross, Li Li, Earl S. Ford, and Simin Liu, "Increased Consumption of Refined Carbohydrates and the Epidemic of Type 2 Diabetes in the United States: an Ecologic Assessment," *Am J Clin Nutr* (May 2004) vol 79 no. 5: 774-779, http://ajcn.nutrition.org/content/79/5/774.full?sid=26ccec59-cbf6-4151-bc7a-883fed38cf4b

[18] Uffe Ravnskov, MD, PhD, *The Cholesterol Myths: Exposing the Fallacy that Saturated Fat and Cholesterol Cause Heart Disease,* (New Trends Publishing Inc., 2000), 49-97.

car as the cholesterol. In a traffic jam, what matters the most? Is it the number of cars that matter or the number of people inside the cars? It is the number of cars (the number of particles that matter).

There are large particle LDLs and small particle LDLs. The small particle causes the most concern, but it is extremely overlooked or not even addressed at all. The small particles get into the arterial walls and oxidize, forming plaque and causing inflammation. This process of oxidation is the main factor in heart disease. The bigger particles do not get into the arterial walls and oxidize. Therefore, the small particles put you at risk for heart disease. The total number of particles, including large and small, can be an indicator of toxicity and is used in the health assessment. When these numbers are out of balance, sugar and bad fats are usually the culprits.

We live in such a fat-phobic society. Look on your grocery shelves and all you see is low-fat this and fat-free that. For the last twenty years, we have been told to avoid saturated fat like the plague. Despite these recommendations, people still gain weight or have trouble losing weight, crave sugar, have decreased energy and enthusiasm, and suffer from a long list of health complications.

Personally and clinically, I have witnessed how increasing good fats has helped people lose weight, gain energy, and reverse chronic symptoms.

You can be overweight and fat deficient. Without the proper fats in your diet, your weight loss and health goals can be a frustrating, uphill battle.

It may be hard to comprehend that you need fat to lose fat. But saturated fat reduces cravings and helps you feel full. You don't feel denied, which is a common problem in many weight loss programs. When you are not eating fat, you fill up with empty calories in foods, such as diet sodas and other fat-free and low-fat products that are loaded with additives and other toxic ingredients, which further deteriorate the body.

"When you consistently use coconut oil (along with other healthy fats), you provide nourishment to every cell in your body, nourishment that supports optimal function of your nerves, brain, hormones, immune system, and metabolism. But beyond that, you trigger a powerful mechanism that is key to success in permanent weight loss: *satiation*."[19]

The dangers of trans fats: Trans fats are an artificially produced fat found widely in processed and packaged foods such as chips, margarine, and baked goods. Trans fats are created when polyunsaturated fats (PUFAs) that normally remain liquid at room temperature are subjected to high temperatures during processing (partial hydrogenation), which makes the liquid behave like a solid. This finished product has a longer shelf life and is commonly used in spreads. This is cheap to make and keeps foods such as chips and cookies from

[19] Dr. Mary Enig and Sally Fallon, *Eat Fat, Lose Fat,* (Penguin Group Inc., 2005), 7.

seeping through the packages and pretty much has an eternal shelf life. Turning a PUFA into a solid is unnatural, and free radicals form. The free radicals make us sick by increasing the small particle LDLs. This is why, in order to reduce chronic cellular inflammation, you must avoid industrially processed soy, corn, or any vegetable oil.

Our government agencies such as the Food and Drug Administration and the American Heart Association have persuaded Americans to increase their intake of these dangerous oils in order to reduce heart disease and to replace butter with margarine. Extensive studies show that partially hydrogenated oils actually increase the risk for heart disease.

"A study published in the American Journal of Public Health concluded that consumption of trans fats by Americans was responsible for more than 30,000 deaths annually from heart disease."[20]

A person who consumes trans fats is more likely to have a compromised immune system, slow healing, hormone imbalance, trouble losing weight, and other health problems than someone who has a diet high in saturated fats from coconut oil and butter.

---

[20] "Fat in Margarine Is Tied to Heart Problems," *The New York Times*, May 16, 1994, http://www.nytimes.com/1994/05/16/us/fat-in-margarine-is-tied-to-heart-problems.html.

"Healthy fats include omega-3 fatty acids (found in cod liver oil, egg yolks, and flax oil), medium chain fats (found in coconut oil, palm kernel oil, and butter), and long-chain saturated fats (found mostly in meat and dairy products). They'll help you lose weight, increase your energy, boost your immunity to illness, and optimize your digestion."[21]

Despite the efforts of Americans to eat a diet low in fat by eliminating red meat and butter, rates of obesity, heart disease, and other inflammatory diseases have drastically increased. So what is causing the increased rates of obesity and heart disease?

Let's discuss the role of whole grains in chronic inflammation. I had a love affair with grains, especially corn and bread. Popular books such as *Wheat Belly* by William Davis, MD and *Grain Brain* by David Perlmutter have made the connection between grains and chronic disease, including infertility, allergies, osteoporosis, depression, dementia, headaches, and anxiety.

---

[21] Dr. Mary Enig and Sally Fallon, *Eat Fat, Lose Fat,* (Penguin Group Inc., 2005), 12.

"The USDA Food Pyramid is based on carbohydrates. The U.S. Department of Agriculture (USDA) Food Pyramid encourages you to eat 6 to 11 servings of grains every day. We're a nation of starch and sugar eaters. This has produced a nation that is either overweight or obese."[22]

The lectins in grains promote inflammation. Lectins are produced by plants as a protective mechanism, similar to the thorns of a cactus. This antinutrient is not readily digested and is resistant to heat. Thirty percent of the foods in our diet are lectin rich. Wheat contains the highly addictive lectin, wheat germ agglutinin, which has been linked with inflammation. Other lectin-containing foods include potatoes, tomatoes, rice, legumes, and meat from grain-fed animals. They are toxic and may trigger symptoms such as headaches, skin problems, and bloating.[23]

Reducing grains played an essential role in normalizing my glucose and insulin levels, as well as losing my weight, clearing my skin, stabilizing my mood, improving my sleep, and eliminating my headaches. Decreasing carbohydrate

---

[22] Loren Cordain, PhD, *The Paleo Diet: Lose Weight and Get Healthy by Eating the Foods You Were Designed to Eat,* (Houghton Mifflin Harcourt, November 29, 2010), Kindle edition.

[23] Sayer Ji, *Opening Pandora's Bread Box: The Critical Role of Wheat Lectin in Human Disease,* accessed October 13, 2014, http://www.greenmedinfo.com/page/opening-pandoras-bread-box-critical-role-wheat-lectin-human-disease.

intake reduced fat that is normally stored and allowed my body to use fat instead of glucose for energy. With the increase of good fats, I noticed that my appetite was satisfied, and many times, I did not feel hungry throughout the day.

The reason why The Cellular Healing Diet is effective is because it includes foods that are low in sugar and rich in good fats and eliminates grains. Food choices include the following:

- Grass-fed beef
- Free-range poultry
- Wild game and wild fish
- Cultured dairy from grass-fed cows
- Fruits and vegetables—preferably organic and locally grown

It is important to avoid the following foods while on the healing program:

- High glycemic fruits such as bananas and mangoes
- Grains such as wheat, rice, and corn
- Legumes such as beans and peanuts

Nutritional Quality of Organic Versus Conventional Fruits, Vegetables, and Grains

"Organic crops contained significantly more vitamin C, iron, magnesium, and phosphorus and significantly less nitrates than conventional crops. There were nonsignificant trends showing less protein but of a better quality and a higher content of nutritionally significant minerals with lower amounts of some heavy metals in organic crops compared to conventional ones.

Conclusions: There appear to be genuine differences in the nutrient content of organic and conventional crops."[24]

I used to be a vegetarian. I was a bad vegetarian, and I made myself sick being a bad vegetarian. Unless you are dedicated to feeding yourself well, you may not get all the nutrients you need. However, I believe being a healthy vegetarian is possible; it takes work. You need to make sure you are getting enough protein in your diet. Protein is usually what's missing in vegetarian diets.

---

[24] Virginia Worthington, "Nutritional Quality of Organic Versus Conventional Fruits, Vegetables, and Grains," *The Journal of Alternative and Complementary Medicine*, 7(2), (April 2001): 161-173. doi:10.1089/107555301750164244.

All Protein Isn't Alike

"Some of the protein you eat contains all the amino acids needed to build new proteins. This kind is called complete protein. Animal sources of protein tend to be complete. Other protein sources lack one or more "essential" amino acids—that is, amino acids that the body can't make from scratch or create by modifying another amino acid. Called incomplete proteins, these usually come from fruits, vegetables, grains, and nuts.

Vegetarians need to be aware of this. To get all the amino acids needed to make new protein—and thus to keep the body's systems in good shape—people who don't eat meat, fish, poultry, eggs, or dairy products should eat a variety of protein-containing foods each day."[25]

Incorporating better choices of meats, fish, vegetables, fruits, nuts, and seeds played a huge part in my treatment plan. The choices of green leafy vegetables, grass-fed meats, and wild fish and game provided me with good, solid protein that encouraged lean, healthy muscle mass.

---

[25] Harvard School of Public Health, "Protein: Moving Closer to Center Stage," accessed October 13, 2014, http://www.hsph.harvard.edu/nutritionsource/protein-full-story/.

Grain-fed beef vs. Grass-fed beef

"Research spanning three decades supports the argument that grass-fed beef (on a g/g fat basis), has a more desirable SFA lipid profile (more C18:0 cholesterol neutral SFA and less C14:0 & C16:0 cholesterol elevating SFAs) as compared to grain-fed beef. Grass-finished beef is also higher in total CLA (C18:2) isomers, TVA (C18:1 t11) and n-3 FAs on a g/g fat basis. This results in a better n-6:n-3 ratio that is preferred by the nutritional community. Grass-fed beef is also higher in precursors for Vitamin A and E and cancer fighting antioxidants such as GT and SOD activity as compared to grain-fed contemporaries."[26]

During the treatment phase, I implemented some of these best practices:

- Shop at local farmers' markets—Shop for fresh, local produce
- Be flexible—Eat soup at breakfast, eat eggs for dinner, and so forth.
- Fast intermittently—Conserve the body's energy and direct it toward healing. There are various methods to

[26] Cynthia A Daley, Amber Abbott, Patrick S Doyle, Glenn A Nader, Stephanie Larson, "A review of fatty acid profiles and antioxidant content in grass-fed and grain-fed beef," *Nutr J.* (2010) 9: 10, published online 2010 March 10, doi: 10.1186/1475-2891-9-10, PMCID: PMC2846864, http://www.nutritionj.com/content/9/1/10.

the intermittent fasting approach. Skipping breakfast and lunch and eating a large dinner at night, fasting twenty-four hours one to three times per week, or a combination of the two. I've incorporated intermittent fasting in my lifestyle and found it to be very beneficial in restoring my health. I used to get real light headed if I didn't eat every two hours, but now my body is an efficient fat burner, and I can go many hours without needing to eat. Studies have shown that intermittent fasting and caloric restriction not only extend your life but also cause hormonal and metabolic changes that aid in weight loss and can ward off heart disease, diabetes, and even cancer. It also downregulates inflammation and helps with hormone sensitivity, the two major causes of most diseases today.[27]

- Customize restaurant meals—Order dishes that emphasize protein and vegetables and not the "prepackaged" specials they commercially prepare. Pass on the bread and the dessert.
- Be prepared—During social eating settings, I will always eat a small meal at home prior to going to the event so that I am not tempted to overindulge. It is also easier to eat healthier food while I am out if I am not really hungry.

---

[27] S. Anton and C. Leeuwenburgh, "Fasting or Caloric Restriction for Healthy Aging," *PubMed Central* 48, no. 10 (2013), accessed October 13, 2014, doi: 10.1016/j.exger.2013.04.011, http://www.ncbi.nlm.nih.gov/pmc/articles/PMC3919445/#__ffn_sectitle.

- Cook the majority of my meals at home—Cook large portions and freeze leftovers. This always ensures that I have something quick on hand to keep from making quick, impulsive decisions that could result in eating an item not on my approved foods list.
- Incorporate burst training—The best type of workout for fat loss! High intensity workout for 20 to 40 seconds followed by 90 to 120 seconds of rest or low impact for recovery, for four to eight cycles (depending on fitness levels). During high intensity, the body is burning stored sugar (glycogen) and burns fat for the next twenty-four to forty-eight hours after the workout to replace glycogen stores. This increases overall metabolism and turns the body from a sugar burner to a fat burner.[28]
- Include supplements—Use a supplemental protocol to improve physiology and encourage cellular detox.

I know I just shared a lot of information that may be foreign or overwhelming to you. Sometimes we fail to take action if we are bombarded with too much information. I want to encourage you to succeed by letting you know it is okay to feel what you are feeling. It is not necessary to figure this out overnight. Remember, it's a journey, and these are more applications you can put in your toolbox. I've been

[28] Stephen H. Boutcher, "High-Intensity Intermittent Exercise and Fat Loss," (2011), accessed October 13,2014, doi: 10.1155/2011/868305

studying health and nutrition for almost twenty years, and I am still learning.

It is not necessary to be 100 percent organic to see results. Choose what you can handle, and incorporate more into your life as you become more confident. For example, you can first focus on eating the right types of foods, and then gradually increase the quality of those foods (grass-fed, organic, and so on) when you can. You can start to eliminate bread or drink more water.

The most compliant and committed patients are the ones who get well the fastest. You have to evaluate your circumstances to determine which actions steps you need to take. We all have different needs, and programs vary from person to person. This is truly the only way you will complete your journey successfully. Gone are the days when you do not dedicate yourself entirely to the task of getting better. You will learn how your present and future choices will affect the quality of your life in the following chapters.

You can keep your goals realistic by asking your doctor or health coach when and how soon to expect results for each area you are working on. He or she will help you estimate the time frames and can tell you when and what to expect at each phase.

Journey Notes:

Based on the general guidance provided in this chapter, list three action steps you can begin *today* that will get you closer to your health care goals.

In the past, what has prevented you from committing or taking action? What can you do to change it? What are the biggest obstacles you believe you will face? (Do you not know how to cook? Do you work long hours? Do you have time or money concerns?)

What motivates you to take action?

Sharing what you're doing with someone you trust is powerful. Who in your circle can be your accountability partner that you share your journey with?

It's important to celebrate your victories! What type of reward system can you set up to acknowledge your wins?

CHAPTER 7

Stage Four: Feeling Discouraged

The best way out is always through.

~ Robert Frost

You have done your best to make all the right decisions up to your point of setback. It seems as if everything started to spiral downward at some point, and you quickly began to focus on your failures and not your successes.

This stage is important to understand, because this is where most of us give up. I believe it would be safe to assume that most of us have felt discouraged at one time or another. We didn't get the job we wanted, so we stopped job hunting. We couldn't fit into our favorite dress, so we threw it out. We couldn't run a mile without stopping, so we figured this wasn't the activity for us. Becoming discouraged also happens when our expectations aren't met. We can all come up with a time we gave up because of unmet expectations. We were hoping to have lost ten pounds in two weeks, and we only lost five.

We've been taking digestive enzymes for a month, and we are still dealing with gas and bloating.

Feeling discouraged can be associated with feelings of hopelessness, confusion, anger, fear, and boredom. Instead of letting these overwhelming emotions defeat you, let's dig deeper and analyze why you may be feeling this way.

I've been at this stage so many times. I tend to be hard on myself, so when things didn't work out as anticipated, I felt like the world was going to end. It felt like, no matter what I did, nothing worked.

Let me share an example of when I first joined a network marketing company. I would get so fired up about the business and would be absolutely sure it was my ticket to financial freedom. I would purchase my business packet and marketing materials and dive right in with my list of prospects. I would be on every conference call, anxious to learn from the best. Initially I would be excited about all the wins I would hear from my team. Some of them would just climb up the ladder seemingly overnight. A month would pass, and I would still be looking for my first team member. I would feel envious and discouraged, wondering why they were doing so well and I was struggling. I was doing my cold calls and introducing the products, but I wasn't going beyond the associate level. I would believe it was the product, move on to another company, and the cycle would continue. I repeated this cycle at least half a dozen times.

Looking back, the reasons why I didn't succeed were because I didn't get in front of enough people and I didn't do follow ups. It wasn't the company that was failing me, it was my fear of rejection. Instead of moving on to the next prospect, I shut down and gave up. This fear of rejection didn't just affect my inability to succeed in any network marketing company. It affected my marriage, my friendships, my practice, and my health.

These inadequacies numb us. We become our own worst enemies, getting involved with self-sabotage. Despite our good intentions, we eventually end up where we started or hit a plateau, unable to get further in life. Willpower and discipline fail us. What now?

The answer lies in our self-limiting beliefs. Our beliefs direct our choices, behaviors, and actions. We need to evaluate those old programs that are running in our minds, preventing us from getting what we want. What are some of the limiting beliefs that have been holding you back? Here are some examples I currently hear or have experienced.

Things never work out for me.
I don't have the money.
I have too much going on.
I am not a morning person.
I don't have enough time.
I will never get ahead.
I am not smart enough.
I am too old.
This is too difficult for me.
I am not good enough.

You feel discouraged when your limiting beliefs start to scream at you. Don't believe the lies! It is possible to change these old programs.

Our behaviors are a direct reflection of our beliefs.

Monitor your thoughts daily, and start to replace those negative, self-limiting beliefs with more affirmative thoughts.

Revisit your why. Are your thoughts congruent with your why? Is your why to have more energy to play with your kids, but you keep telling yourself you are tired? Once you become more aware of your thoughts, you may be surprised at the things you habitually say to yourself.

When that self-limiting belief pops in your head, cancel it right away and replace it with a more positive statement. For example, if "I am always tired!" comes up, think about what it would feel like to have an abundance of energy. What would you do with that energy? Play with your kids, clean the house, or visit a close friend? Visualize as though it is happening right now. Create a new statement, such as, "My body is getting stronger every day!" It's amazing how your body quickly responds to the new thought. It takes practice. But once you start to master it, watch your life and your health change. There are many effective techniques and there is research about how our beliefs control our biology.[29]

---

[29] Bruce H. Lipton, PhD, *The Biology of Belief: Unleashing the Power of Consciousness, Matter & Miracles*, (Hay House, 2005).

Your beliefs become your thoughts
Your thoughts become your words
Your words become your actions
Your actions become your habits
Your habits become your values
Your values become your destiny

-Mahatma Gandhi

Success and personal growth come from being aware of your beliefs and taking responsibility for your actions. You must not confuse your struggles with failure. Look at your struggles as a test, a chance to assess and reevaluate. Instead of giving up when things get tough, this is the best time to reflect on why this is occurring, strap on your boots, and do your best to get through it. Most of my disappointments have come from giving up too soon, and most of my successful moments come after I have gone through the struggle. Sometimes what you see on the other side of the struggle is better than what you ever imagined.

I have found this stage to be where I learned the most about myself and what I am capable of. I now welcome challenges, and instead of believing that they came up to defeat me, I take them on, knowing that something rewarding is on the other side.

In my healing journey, I momentarily gave up because of

discouragement and lack of enthusiasm. When I first started The Cellular Healing Diet and had to give up my favorite food, bread, in order balance my sugar levels, I lost almost twenty pounds in the first six months. I was ecstatic! Then for the next three months, the weight wasn't changing at all. I thought I was on to something and had cracked the code, only to remain stuck for months. My self-limiting thought was *it is hard to lose weight after forty.* Then I started to go back to why I started in the first place. I began to see myself at my ideal weight. I began to feel the abundance of energy I had. I continued to immerse myself in learning about health, listen to audio, read books, hang around like-minded people, and go to the gym. I had to feed my mind with what I wanted and to cancel what I didn't. You can't think a positive thought and a negative thought at the same time.

Once I achieved one goal, I moved on to the next one and readjusted my program when necessary. For example, when I was 205 pounds, my first goal was to get under 200. When I hit 199 my next goal was to get to the 180s. It is so much more manageable to set up smaller goals and celebrate your successes along the way. Stay focused on the journey instead of the outcome. Refuse to beat yourself up if you find yourself off track. Just stop and evaluate your thoughts.

Occasionally, we want to return to our old habits because they were more "comfortable." We remember how much easier it was to go to the drive-through versus cooking a whole meal. That's human nature. The good news is you can create new habits. This is the time to be creative. Reach out to others who are doing similar things and share ideas. That's why I encourage a friend or a health coach to go through this journey with you.

You may experience being so overwhelmed from making the changes to eating healthier foods. You may find it's been especially hard to get the bread out of your diet. Plus, you may get discouraged when you get on the scale and it hasn't budged in two weeks.

I understand, and I know it is not easy. It is very normal to feel this way when you are doing something new. In this stage, you begin to want to give up, and unfortunately, most people do. This is when you have to remember your why, your purpose for wanting to get well. Ask yourself if it is still worth it.

In my early years of practice, I didn't recognize when patients were going through this stage. We all go through this cycle of challenges. It's actually a part of your growth in this new process of a healthier lifestyle. Don't look at it as failure.

We live in a culture where we want things fast and easy. And if we don't get them in that fashion, they're not worth having. This is in a lot of aspects of our lives, not just in healing. People just don't want to wait anymore and assume that whatever they are doing is not working. You are getting better, and you have already come a long way. Just because you don't see the major changes every day doesn't mean they are not there. Remember, you are healing at a cellular level, and you may be dealing with some chronic issues you have been living with for decades. Healing takes time, and you are not alone.

The fact that you are reading this book is proof enough that you are dedicated to this process. Your frustration is the anger you feel because you are anxious to succeed in this endeavor, and it means a lot to you. Some people fail to reach out or acknowledge that they are struggling. Some people have dropped out all together at this point without confronting the issue. The fact that you are confessing your challenges and your setbacks is powerful! Together we will get you through this. In the long run, this will make you stronger and more confident. You will look back at this moment one day and realize how far you have really come.

Evaluate your progress, and appreciate the changes you have made so far. Continue to log all your foods and beverages, even when you do not make the healthiest choices. Be strong when you start to feel overwhelmed at your attempts to include healthy choices for you and your family, staying up at night to prepare those meals and stopping by the grocery store to pick up items. That is not an easy feat, and you should really be proud of what you have achieved so far. Talk to a friend or coach. Don't complain about your struggle, be proactive, and seek a tangible solution that will get you back on track.

This is what striving for success feels like. It is normal to have good and bad days. I find myself thinking of one of my favorite quotes by Greg Behrendt: "Life's biggest rewards come from the biggest challenges."

It's important not to be hard on yourself. Don't give up.

Continue to be more patient with the process. And if you do slip up, don't let it defeat you.

New habits are hard to form at first, but they will get easier; I promise. In your journey, focus on what you have achieved so far, such as the energy you have gained, the weight you have lost, or the soundness of your sleep. It is important to focus on the positives and not dwell on the negatives. Be proud of what you have accomplished so far.

The point here is to learn from your mistakes. It is okay to make them as long as you learn from them. Don't make the error of believing that your mistakes are a sign of failure. Mistakes do not have to be setbacks that destroy your journey. Take a mistake for what it is. A mistake! It is not the end of the world. This is when you sit back to reevaluate, reassess, and move forward.

Stage four, feeling discouraged, is not permanent. Don't make it an opportunity to give up. Your breakthrough may be right around the corner.

Stop and take a deep breath. This is the reason why I utilize the health-coaching format. Because when my patients start to slack, that's really when they need the most support. If the strong commitment is there, they are able to get back on their own two feet. It is often required to revisit their why and their wins.

Here are four steps that will help you move forward despite the struggles you face.

1. Organize your time. This is the most simple and overlooked step. Plan your days by keeping a calendar of your daily and weekly tasks and checking them off as you complete each one. When you have not completed something, take a moment to evaluate the reasons, and then work on a resolution to make it happen. Is it something you didn't do because of something else? Or was it mismanaged planning that caused you to not do it? Is the task important? Will it bring you closer to your goals?

   Many of us claim to be too busy, but when you put this into practice, you will really begin to realize that a lot of your time is wasted on things that are not productive. The most common time wasters are social media, browsing the internet, and watching reality TV. You have the power and capability to change the circumstances to result in a positive outcome. Use your time wisely!

2. Monitor your thoughts. Envision every day why you are making changes. This daily reminder of why you are making lifestyle changes will motivate you and reinforce the importance of sticking to your goals. Keep your why in front of you.

3. Work on becoming consistent. Consistency turns into a natural flow of working your plan each day without hesitation. You start to develop new habits that work

for you instead of against you. It will be very difficult to reach any destination if you keep looking backward. Trust in the process, and keep moving forward.

4. Surround yourself with positive and supportive people. Have an accountability partner. Having a positive support team keeps you on track. Take note and celebrate the positive changes in your life. Celebrate with your team. Dwelling on the negatives will only hold you back. There is so much to be thankful for. Focus on those.

It is important to realize that as long as you are doing the right things and taking consistent steps in the right direction, you will get well. The road to success is not a straight line. Sometimes you fall off track, just to get back on again. It does get easier. You are eating much better than you were before. No, you are not perfect, but you are better than yesterday. Hold on to those positive wins. Once you manage to adopt a new idea, move on to the next one. Trust me, you will never run out of things to learn, and there is *always* room for improvement. Every step matters. It doesn't matter how small.

Journey Notes:

List at least three limiting beliefs that tend to come up most frequently when you are ready to give up (for example, not enough energy or not enough time).

Now observe each of your excuses, and replace them with solutions that will push you forward.

List at least three wins that have occurred in your life in the last six months.

What did you overcome to experience those wins?

CHAPTER 8

Stage 5: Freedom

How you do anything is how you do everything.
~ T. Harv Eker

You have been reflecting on how far you have really come. What a ride: the frustration, the challenges, the tears, the discouragement, and the growth.

Not only do I have my health, I feel a different clarity, an inner strength. I feel like I can do anything! I have a deeper purpose in my life. I feel alive!

I still enjoy my life as a doctor-advisor-health coach. I have found more balance and fun in my life. There is inner peace that resides in me. I am able to face challenges head on.

I enjoy sharing what I went through and encouraging others to do the same. We have so much stacked against us in today's world, but if I can create more love and health, then I am with it.

Every day, my mission it to be better than I was yesterday. I am able to forgive myself for the past mistakes I've made. My experiences help me appreciate where I am today. This is my journey. Life is a journey. I won't stop. There is always room for more … for better.

At this stage in the game, you are doing it! Acknowledge what you've achieved. No matter how big or small, it's time to dance! Shout! Celebrate! What a journey!

This is the stage where friends and family have noticed your progress. They have noticed your glowing skin and shining confidence and have told you how great you look and how happy you seem. They are curious to know more of what you are doing.

You have placed *you* at the front of the line, and it feels wonderful!

This is where we all want to end up. I live to hear these types of testimonials. In my personal testimony, I had managed to lose a total of seventy pounds from my heaviest weight. My personal journey helped me find a way to help others get their lives back. I worked hard and invested in my health. I am still working on different aspects of my health. For example, at the time of writing this book, I am detoxing heavy metals, such as lead and mercury from my body. I will continue to work on my health and improve my programs to help others.

I feel fantastic, and it is an honor to see others find freedom in their health and their lives. In my practice, I've seen many struggles and tears, but when you get to this phase, you look back and say, "It was worth it!" Those struggles build your faith, and those setbacks build your confidence. You become stronger through it all, and you know what, another journey awaits. It's usually something greater, maybe even more challenging. But you've been through the stages before, and you will go through them again and again.

This empowerment gets you to the point that you want to share your story. Your story can be a turning point in someone else's life.

Now that you are seeing fabulous results and feeling absolutely wonderful, how do you stay on this path? You have put in the hard work, followed all the steps, and had setbacks but have overcome them—now what?

Here are two tips to keep you on your journey:

1. Keep your commitments and stay consistent

I've already told you how important consistency is. At this stage, it is still vital to your progress and to maintaining what you have already accomplished. The steps got you to this point, and those same steps will keep you here.

On those occasions when things don't work out as planned (and it will happen), keep in mind that a bump in the road is not a setback; it's a bump in the road. When it occurs, be flexible, adjust your route, and keep going!

2. Keep your vision in front of you

Progress has not just happened by accident. You have made some major strides. Once you achieve one major goal, you will find that another one awaits. Continue maintaining a daily journal and writing down your vision for the next thirty days, sixty days, ninety days, one year, five years, and so forth. This will be the best reinforcement toward continued success.

Collect images that inspire you, write words of encouragement, and post pictures of yourself to monitor your continued progress. It is invaluable when you can look back over the images you have created for yourself during your journey. You will soon realize that along your journey, it's beyond weight loss or getting out of pain; it's also about being more joyful and content. You begin to discover more about yourself and your own true power and about how you can help and serve others. It is possible to be free in health! Live the best days and moments of your life right now!

You have finally had a breakthrough. But, it doesn't mean it is over. You have built the inner muscle to take on the next journey. You have reached a certain point only to realize that there is something better in store! The challenges may get bigger, but you are confident that you can handle them. This is what life is all about. I am excited to be a part of it!

Journey Notes:

What has been your latest breakthrough?
What occasion have you used your experience to help others?
What have you learned about yourself?
What does freedom mean to you?
Do you have a new why? If so, what is it?

APPENDIX A

A Brief Description of Blood Chemistry Markers

These are some of the most common markers you should become familiar with.

GGT (Gamma-Glutamyl Transpeptidase)

This test determines liver cell dysfunction and detects alcohol-induced liver disease. GGT is elevated in all forms of liver disease.

AST (Aspartate Transaminase)

AST levels rise as a result of any injury or death of the cells that are present in the heart, liver, skeletal muscle, kidney, brain, pancreas, spleen, and lungs.

ALT (Alanine Aminotransferase)

An enzyme found in high concentrations in the liver. ALT increases with liver dysfunction.

Glucose

Glycogen is the storage form of carbohydrates that converts to glucose in the liver. Glucose is increased in insulin resistance, diabetes, and liver failure.

Hemoglobin A1C

Measure of blood glucose concentration. HbA1C is not influenced by daily fluctuations in blood glucose concentration, but it does depend on the blood glucose concentration.

Triglycerides

A lipid found in the blood. Increased triglycerides are commonly associated with total cholesterol elevation. Sources of triglycerides include the diet and liver.

Alk. Phos. (Alkaline Phosphatase)

An enzyme that mainly originates in the liver, bone and placenta. This factor is normally elevated in children and teens. This test is an index of bone and liver disease.

Cholesterol

Found in animal oils and fats and is an essential component of cell membrane development and sex hormones. Total cholesterol includes HDL-C and LDL-C. Cholesterol is needed by every cell in the body.

HDL-C (High-density Lipoproteins)

Plays a role in cholesterol and lipid transport from the peripheral tissues to the liver.

LDL-C (Low-density Lipoproteins)

Plays a role in cholesterol and lipid transport from the liver to the peripheral tissues.

LDL-P

The total number of LDL particles (large and small). Particles transport cholesterol throughout the body.

Small LDL-P

A measure of the small LDL particles. Smaller particles oxidize more and are more likely to penetrate in the endothelium. This is a strong indicator for heart disease.

TG/HDL Ratio

A very accurate predictor of heart disease, oxidized small particles, and insulin resistance.

For more tools and resources that will help you along your healing journey, please visit www.DrLeona.com.